CONTENT

1

MANAGEMENT OF DISCOLOURED ATERIOR TEETH BY DIRECT COMPOSITE VENEERS

PATIENT NAME – Deepak

AGE/SEX – 20 Yrs/ Male

CHIEF COMPLAINT – Patient complains of discoloured teeth in upper right and left front tooth region of mouth since 10 years

HISTORY OF PRESENT ILLNESS – Patient gives a history of discoloured teeth in maxillary anterior tooth region of mouth since 10 years.

INTRA-ORAL EXAMINATION – Fluorosis irt 11, 12, 13, 14, 21, 22 ,23, 24

FINAL DIAGNOSIS – Dental fluorosis irt 11, 12, 13, 14, 21, 22 ,23, 24

TREATMENT PLAN – Direct composite veneers irt 11, 12, 13, 14, 21, 22, 23, 24

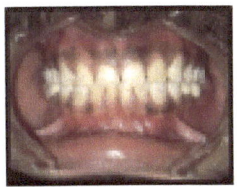

PRE OPERATIVE

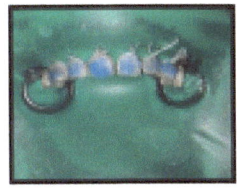

ACID ETCHING

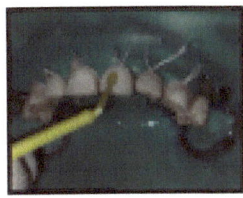

APPLICATION OF BONDING AGENT

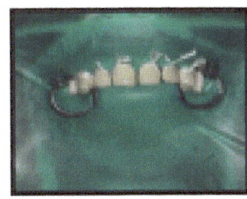

PLACEMENT OF COMPOSITE

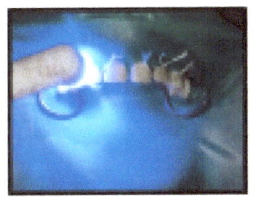

LIGHT ACTIVATION

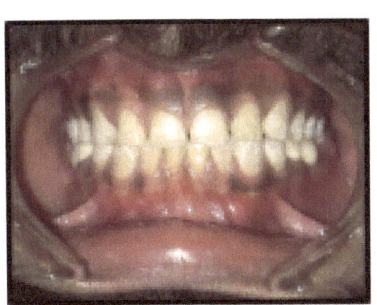
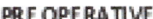

PRE OPERATIVE

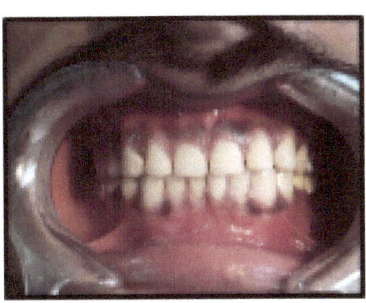

POST OPERATIVE

2

MANAGEMENT OF COMPLICATED CROWN FRACTURE OF MAXILLARY RIGHT CENTRAL INCISOR BY REATTACHMENT USING FIBER POST

PATIENT NAME – Rajani

AGE/SEX – 26 Yrs/ Female

CHIEF COMPLAINT – Patient complains of broken tooth in upper front teeth region since 1 day.

HISTORY OF PRESENT ILLNESS – Patient gives a history of trauma 1 day ago.

INTRA-ORAL EXAMINATION – Ellis Class III fracture irt 21

FINAL DIAGNOSIS – Ellis Class III fracture irt 21

TREATMENT PLAN – Root canal therapy followed by reattachment using fiber post irt 21

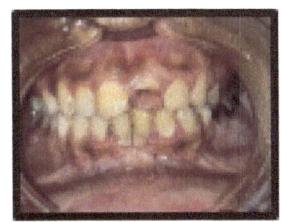
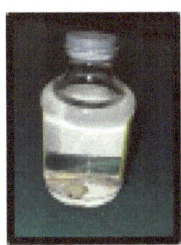
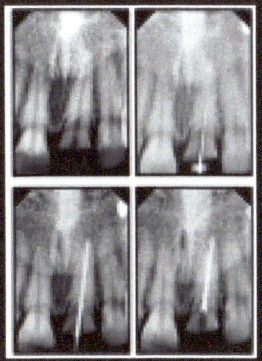

PRE OPERATIVE   FRAGMENT STORED IN NORMAL SALINE   RCT

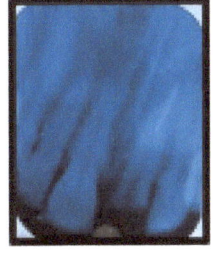
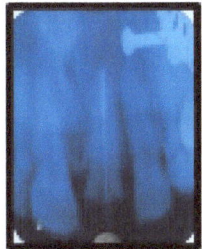
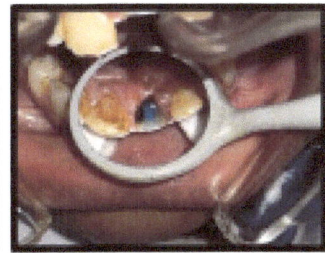

POST SPACE   FIBER POST FIT CHECK   ETCHANT APPLICATION IN POST SPACE

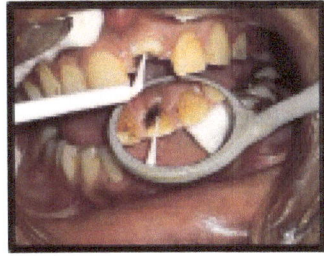
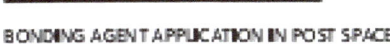
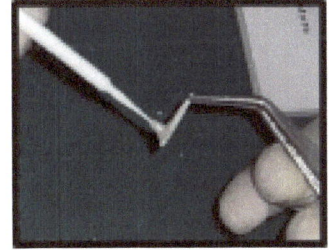

BONDING AGENT APPLICATION IN POST SPACE   DUAL CORE RESIN CEMENT
                                                  PLACED ON FIBER POST

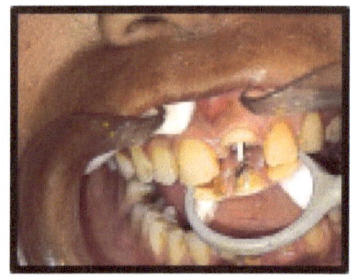

FIBER POST PLACED IN POST SPACE

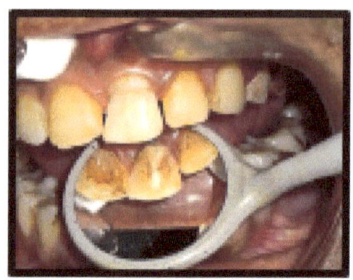

HOLE MADE THROUGH THE PAATAL SURFACE

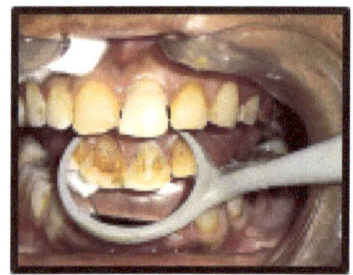

FRAGMENT ATTACHED

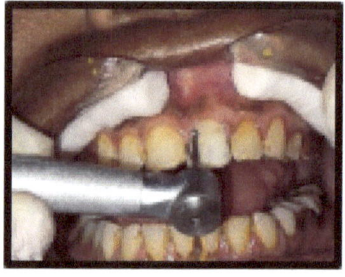

GROOVE MADE ON FRACTURE LINE

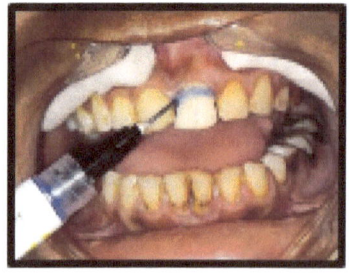

ETCHANT APPLICATION

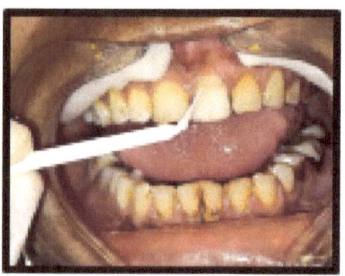

BONDING AGENT APPICATION

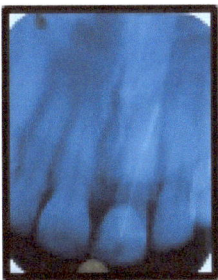

POST OPERATIVE

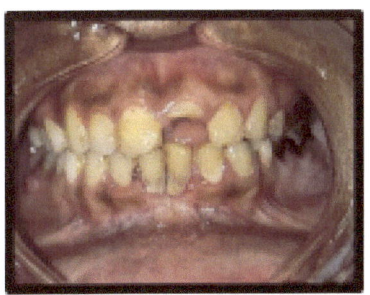
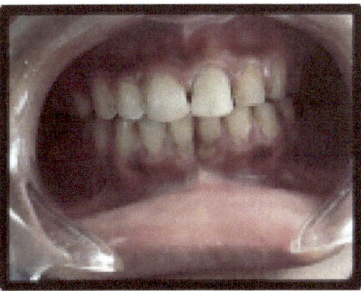

PRE OPERATIVE   POST OPERATIVE

3

MANAGEMENT OF UNCOMPLICATED CROWN FRACTURE OF MAXILLARY RIGHT CENTRAL INCISOR BY REATTACHMENT

PATIENT NAME – Priya

AGE/SEX – 21 Yrs/ Female

CHIEF COMPLAINT – Patient complains of broken tooth in upper front teeth region since 1 day.

HISTORY OF PRESENT ILLNESS – Patient gives a history of trauma 1 day ago.

INTRA-ORAL EXAMINATION – Ellis Class II fracture irt 11

FINAL DIAGNOSIS – Ellis Class II fracture irt 11

TREATMENT PLAN – Fragment reattachment irt 11

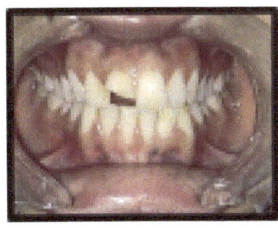

PRE OPERATIVE

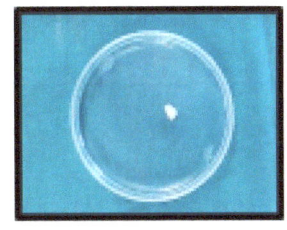

FRAGMENT STORED IN 50% DEXTROSE SOLUTION

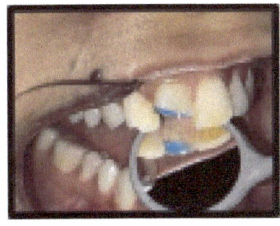

ETCHANT APPLICATION

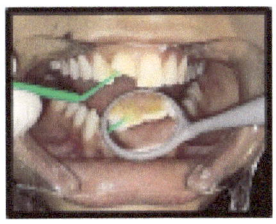

BONDING AGENT APPLICATION

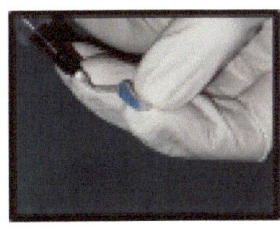

ETCHANT APPLICATION ON TOOTH FRAGMENT

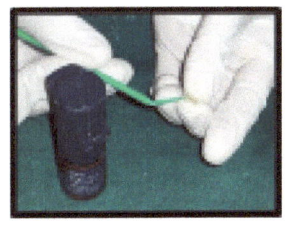

BONDING AGENT APPLICATION ON TOOTH FRAGMENT

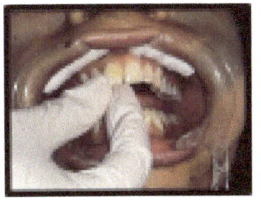

FRAGMENT PLACED IN POSITION WITH FLOWABLE COMPOSITE RESIN

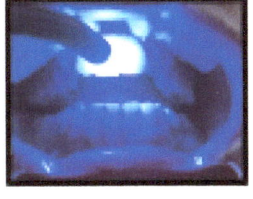

LIGHT ACTIVATION

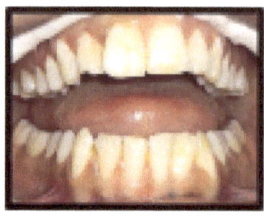

FRAGMENT ATTACHED

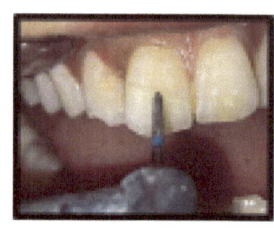

GROOVE MADE ON THE FRACTURE LINE WITH
TORPEDO DIAMOND BUR

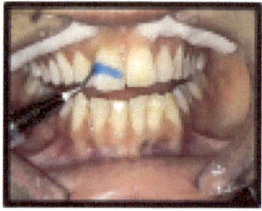

ETCHANT APPLICATION

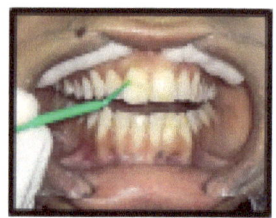

BONDING AGENT APPLICATION

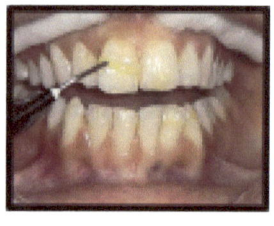

APPLICATION OF FLOWABLE COMPOSITE RESIN IN GROOVE

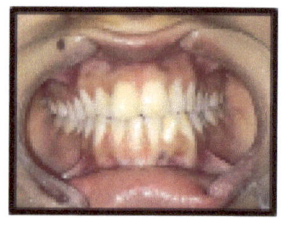

POST OPERATIVE

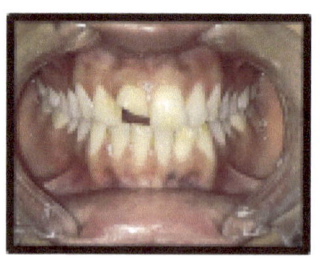

PRE OPERATIVE

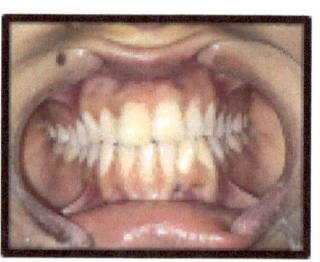

POST OPERATIVE

4

AESTHETIC MANAGEMENT OF DIASTEMA IN MAXILLARY INCISORS BY EMAX CROWNS

PATIENT NAME – Pallavi

AGE/SEX – 40 Yrs/ Female

CHIEF COMPLAINT – Patient complains of gap in upper front tooth region since 20 years.

HISTORY OF PRESENT ILLNESS – Patient complains of gap in upper front tooth region 20 years.

INTRA-ORAL EXAMINATION – Diastema irt 13,12,11,21,22,23

TREATMENT PLAN – Diastema closure by Emax crowns irt 13,12,11,21,22,23

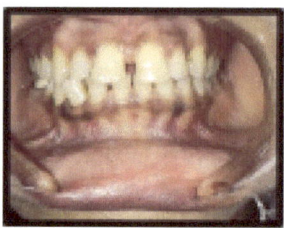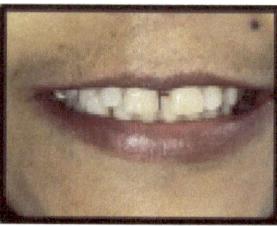

PRE OPERATIVE

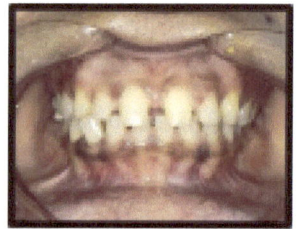

CROWN PREPARATION

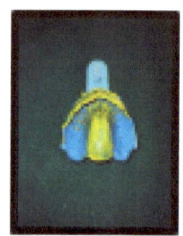

IMPRESSION

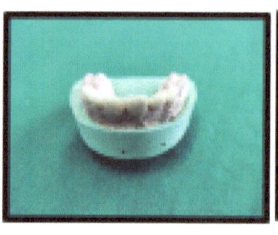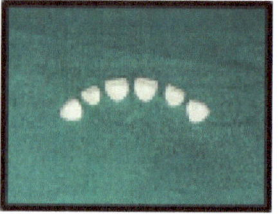

E MAX CROWNS

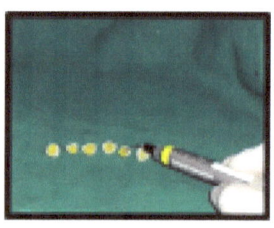

HF ETCHING

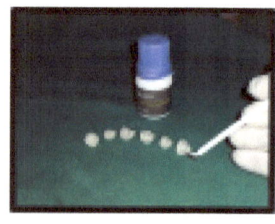

SILANE APPICATION

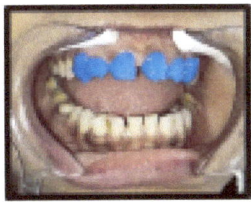

ETCHANT APPLICATION

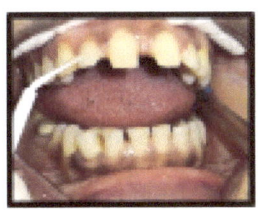

BONDING AGENT

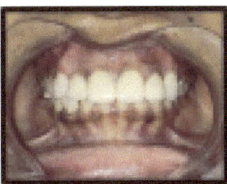
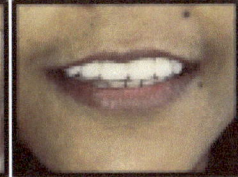

POST OPERATIVE

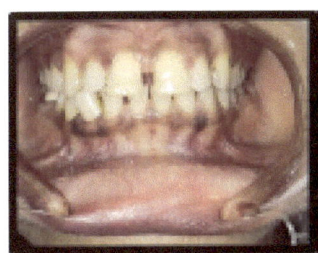
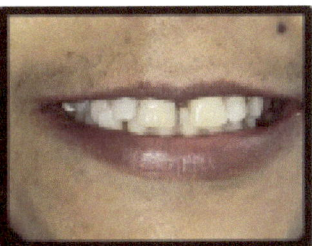

PRE OPERATIVE

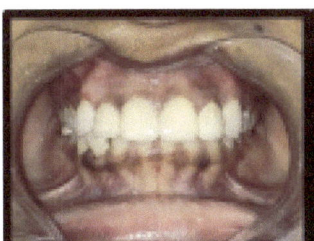
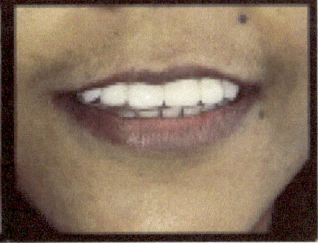

POST OPERATIVE

5

MANAGEMENT OF DISTALLY LUXATED LEFT MAXILLARY CENTRAL INCISOR AND INTRUDED LEFT MAXILLARY CANINE BY INTENTIONAL REPLANTATION AND EXTRUSION FOLLOWED BY LABIAL AND LINGUAL SPLINTING AND ENDODONTIC TREATMENT

PATIENT NAME – Vimal

AGE/SEX – 16 Yrs/ Male

CHIEF COMPLAINT – Patient complains of broken tooth in upper front teeth region since 4 days.

HISTORY OF PRESENT ILLNESS – Patient gives a history of trauma 4 days ago.

INTRA-ORAL EXAMINATION – Lateral luxation irt 21, avulsion irt 22, intrusive luxation irt 23

FINAL DIAGNOSIS – Lateral luxation irt 21, avulsion irt 22, intrusive luxation irt 23

TREATMENT PLAN – Splinting (labial & palatal splint) and Root canal therapy irt 21,23

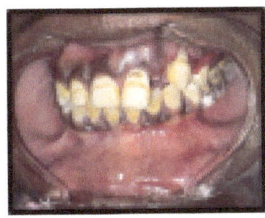

PRE OPERATIVE

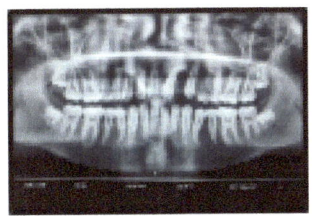

PRE OPERATIVE OPG

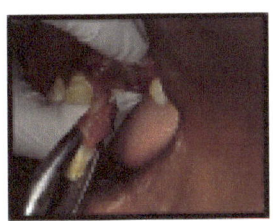

ATRAUMATIC REMOVAL irt 21

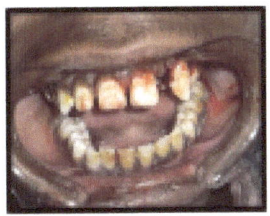

INTENTIONAL REPLANTATION irt 21;
SURGICAL EXTRUSION irt 23

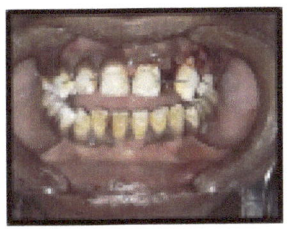

LABIAL SPLINT

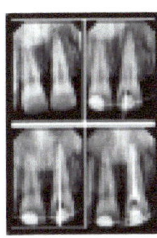

RCT irt 21

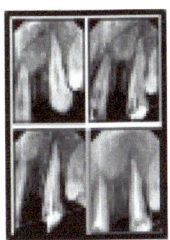

RCT irt 23

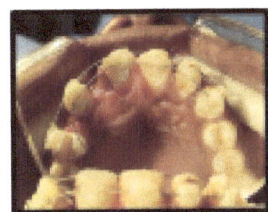

LABIAL & PALATAL SPLINT

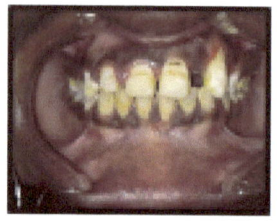

SPLINTS REMOVED AFTER 4 WEEKS

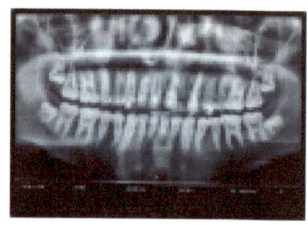

OPG AFTER 4 WEEKS OF SPLINTING

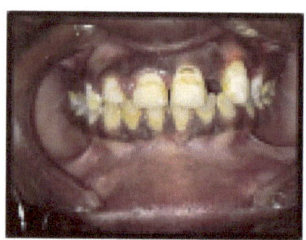

8 WEEKS FOLLOW UP

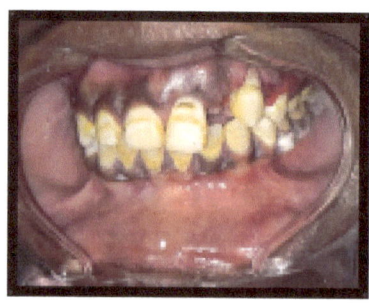

PRE OPERATIVE

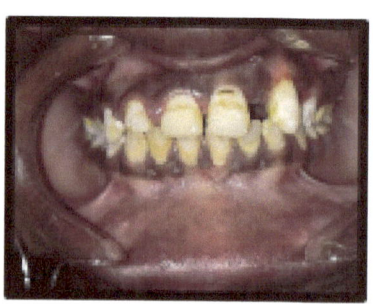

POST OPERATIVE

6

ESTHETIC REHABLITATION OF TRAUMATICALLY INJURED MAXILLARY CENTRAL INCISOR BY ROOT CANAL TREATMENT FOLLOWED BY NON VITAL BLEACHING

PATIENT NAME – Ajay

AGE/SEX – 20 Yrs/ Male

CHIEF COMPLAINT – Patient complains of discoloured teeth in upper front tooth region since 1 year.

HISTORY OF PRESENT ILLNESS – Patient gives a history of trauma 1 year ago.

INTRA-ORAL EXAMINATION – Ellis class IV fracture irt 11

FINAL DIAGNOSIS – Elis class IV fracture irt 11

TREATMENT PLAN – Root canal treatment followed by intra-coronal (non-vital)bleaching irt 11

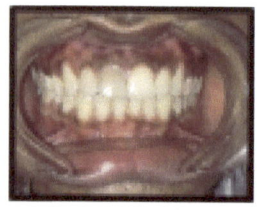

PRE OPERATIVE

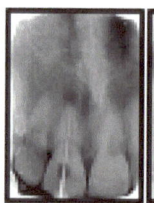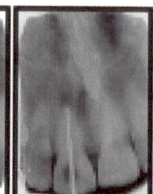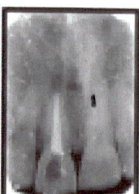

ROOT CANAL THERAPY OF 11

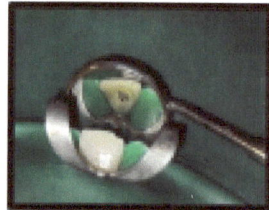

INTRACORONAL CHAMBER

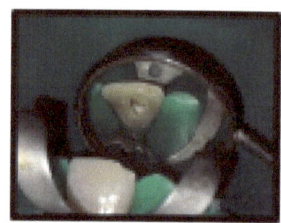

GIC BARRIER

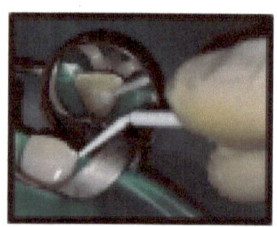

PLACEMENT OF BLEACHING AGENT

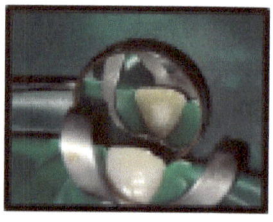

BLEACHING AGENT

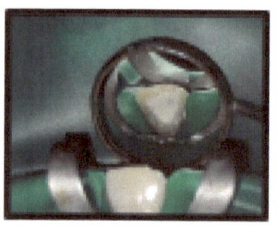

GIC RESTORATION

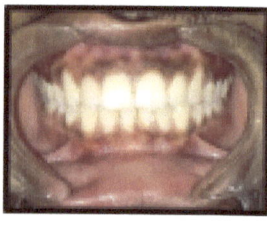

POST OPERATIVE

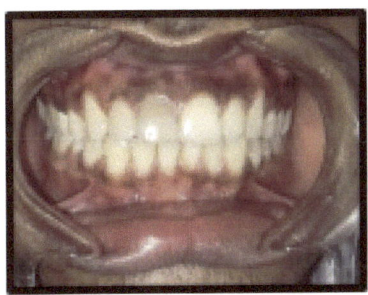 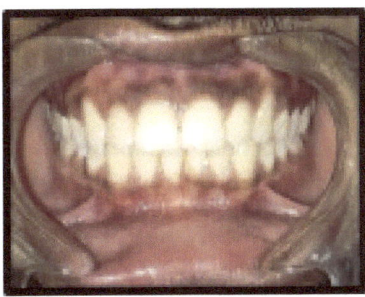

PRE OPERATIVE   POST OPERATIVE

7

MANAGEMENT OF ANTERIOR TEETH WITH FLOUROSIS BY INOFFICE VITAL BLEACHING

PATIENT NAME – Chandrabhan

AGE/SEX – 28 Yrs/ Male

CHIEF COMPLAINT – Patient complains of discoloured teeth in upper right and left front tooth region of mouth since 5 years

HISTORY OF PRESENT ILLNESS – Patient gives a history of discoloured teeth in maxillary anterior tooth region of mouth since 5 years.

INTRA-ORAL EXAMINATION – Generalized fluorosis

FINAL DIAGNOSIS – Dental fluorosis

TREATMENT PLAN – In office vital bleaching

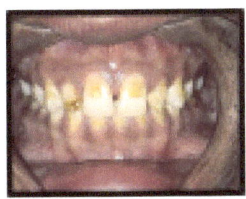

PRE OPERATIVE

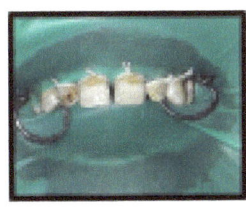

RUBBER DAM APPLICATION

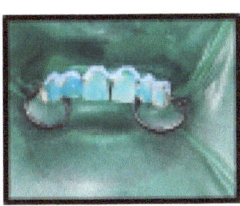

BLEACHING AGENT

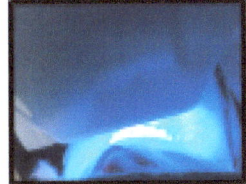

LIGHT ACTIVATION

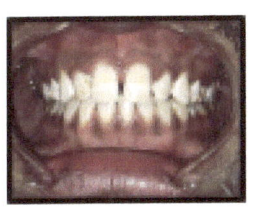

POST OPERATIVE

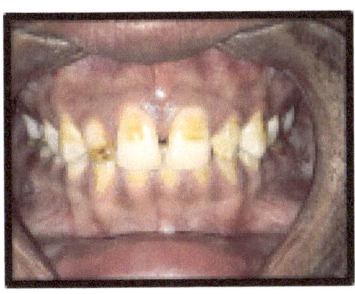

PRE OPERATIVE

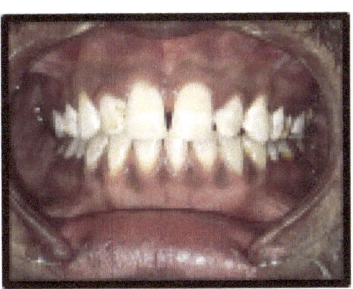

POST OPERATIVE

8

ESTHETIC REHABLITATION OF TRAUMATICALLY INJURED RIGHT AND LEFT MAXILLARY CENTRAL INCISORS BY E MAX CROWN

PATIENT NAME – Sachin Choudhary

AGE/SEX – 16 Yrs/ Male

CHIEF COMPLAINT – Patient complains of broken teeth in upper front tooth region since 1 year.

HISTORY OF PRESENT ILLNESS – Patient gives a history of trauma 1 year ago.

INTRA-ORAL EXAMINATION – Ellis class II fracture irt 11, 21

FINAL DIAGNOSIS – Elis class II fracture irt 11,21

TREATMENT PLAN – Root canal treatment followed by Emax crown irt 11,21

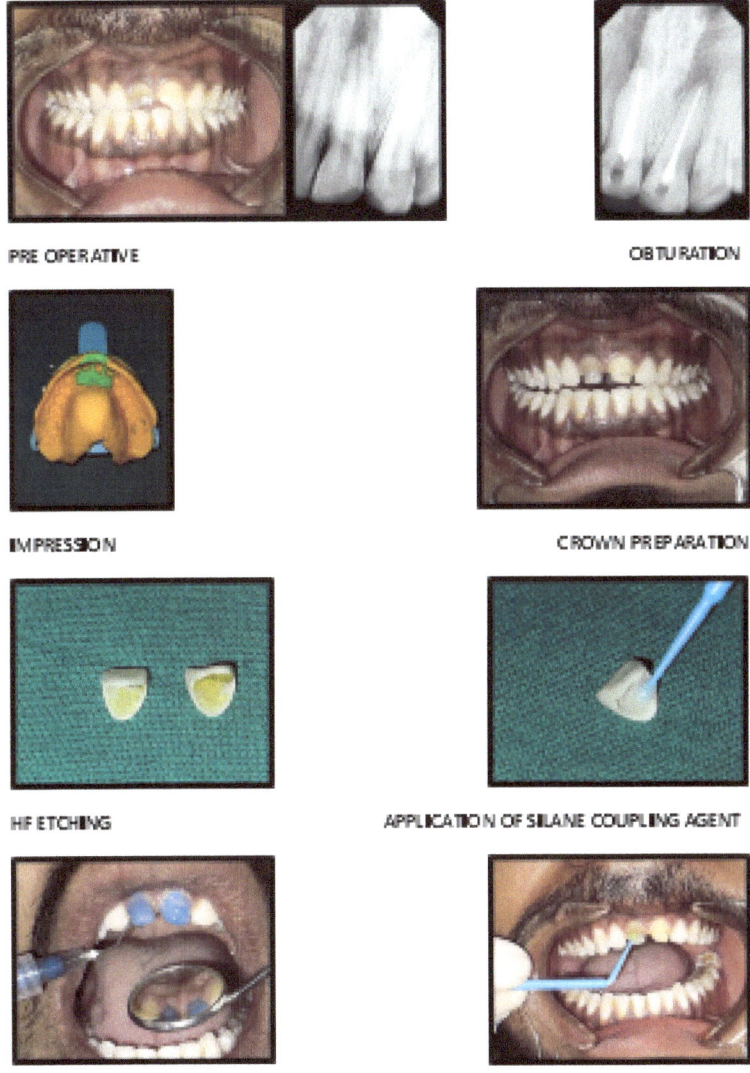

PRE OPERATIVE

OBTURATION

IMPRESSION

CROWN PREPARATION

HF ETCHING

APPLICATION OF SILANE COUPLING AGENT

ETCHING

APPLICATION OF BONDING AGENT

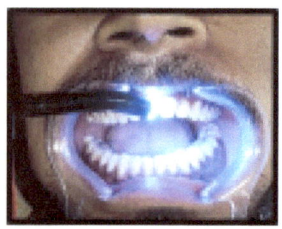

LIGHT ACTIVATION

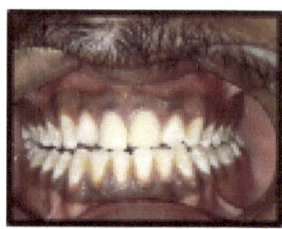

POST OPERATIVE

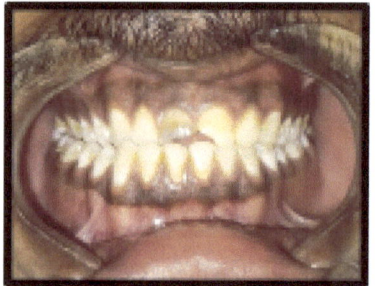

PRE OPERATIVE

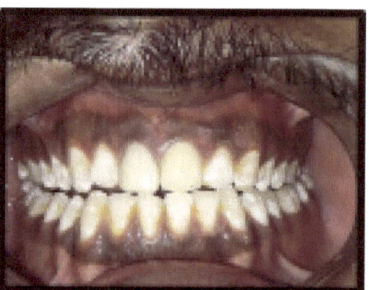

POST OPERATIVE

9

MANAGEMENT OF CLASS II DENTAL CARIES IN MANDIBULAR LEFT SECOND MOLAR WITH MOD INLAY

PATIENT NAME – Manendar

AGE/SEX – 55 Yrs/ Male

CHIEF COMPLAINT – Patient complains of broken filling and food lodgement in lower left back tooth region since 1 month.

HISTORY OF PRESENT ILLNESS – Patient gives a history of filling in same tooth 5 months ago.

INTRA-ORAL EXAMINATION – Faulty restoration irt 36

FINAL DIAGNOSIS – Faulty restoration irt 36

TREATMENT PLAN – MOD Inlay irt 36

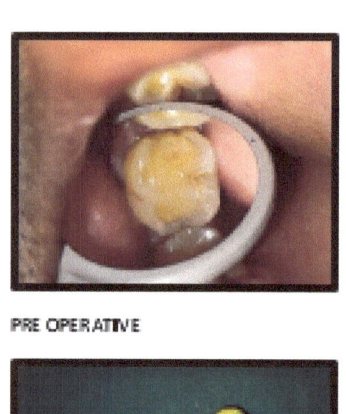

PRE OPERATIVE

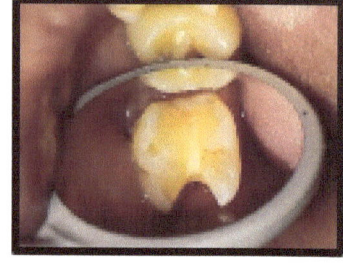
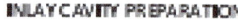

INLAY CAVITY PREPARATION

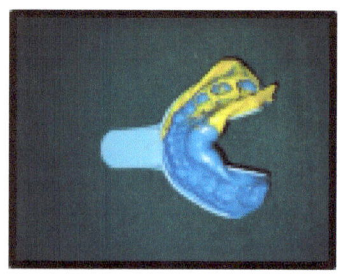

IMPRESSION

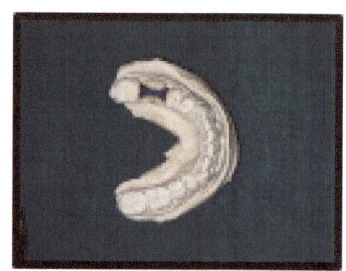

INLAY WAXPATTERN

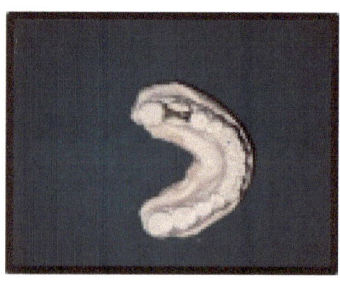

MOD INLAY

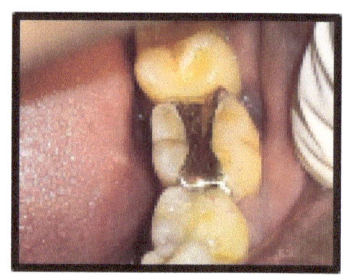

POST OPERATIVE

10

ESTHETIC MANAGEMENT OF ROOT CANAL TREATED MANDIBULAR RIGHT SECOND PREMOLAR WITH SHARONLAY

PATIENT NAME – Rangeeta

AGE/SEX – 40 Yrs/ Female

CHIEF COMPLAINT – Patient complains of broken tooth and food lodgement in lower right back tooth region since 1 month.

HISTORY OF PRESENT ILLNESS – Patient gives a history of RCT and crown in same tooth 5 months ago.

INTRA-ORAL EXAMINATION – Dislodged restoration irt 46

FINAL DIAGNOSIS – Dislodged restoration irt 46

TREATMENT PLAN – Sharonlay irt 46

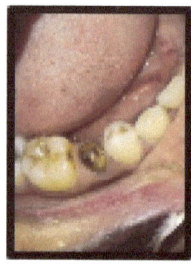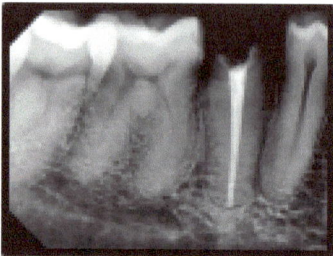

PRE OPERATIVE

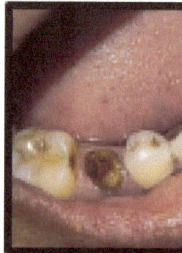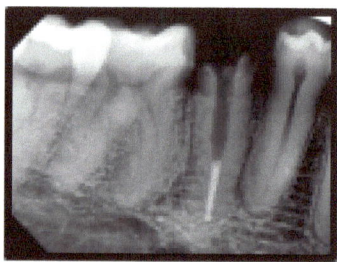

POST SPACE PREPARED

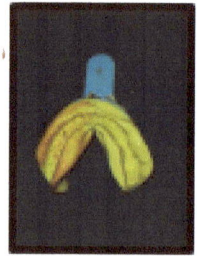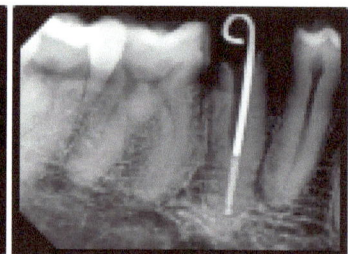

IMPRESSION

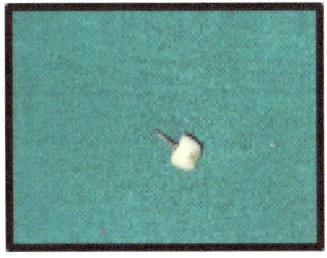

SHARONLAY

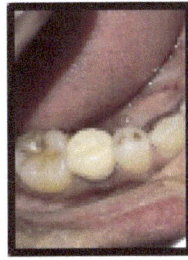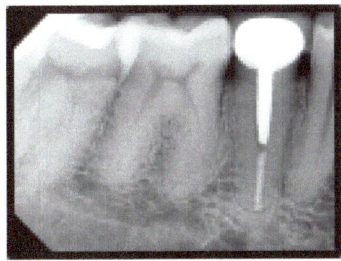

POST OPERATIVE

11

ESTHETIC MANAGEMENT OF ELLIS CLASS II FRACTURE USING PUTTY INDEX

PATIENT NAME – Hemanth

AGE/SEX – 19 Yrs/ Male

CHIEF COMPLAINT – Patient complains of broken tooth in upper front tooth region since 1 year.

HISTORY OF PRESENT ILLNESS – Patient gives a history of trauma 1 year ago.

INTRA-ORAL EXAMINATION – Ellis Class II fracture irt 21

FINAL DIAGNOSIS – Ellis Class II fracture irt 21

TREATMENT PLAN – Compostie restoration irt 21

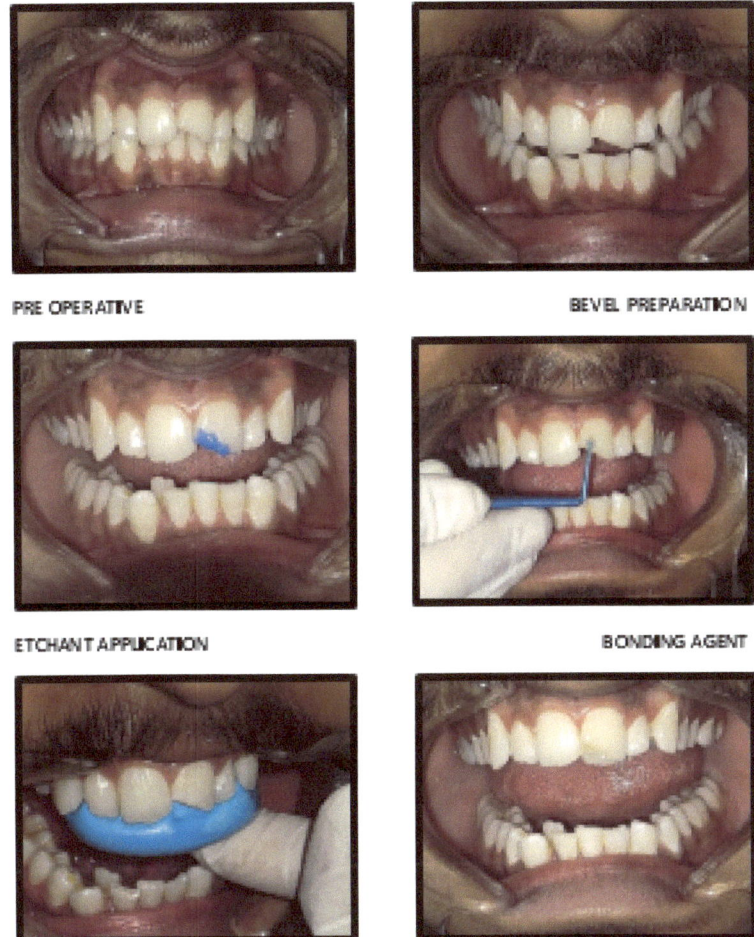

PRE OPERATIVE

BEVEL PREPARATION

ETCHANT APPLICATION

BONDING AGENT

PUTTY INDEX

PALATAL SHELL

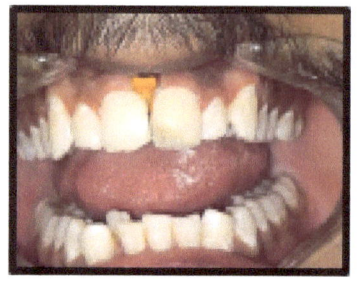

MESIAL WALL BUILD UP

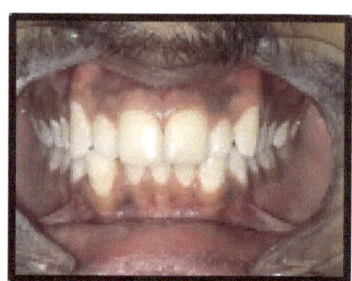

POST OPERATIVE

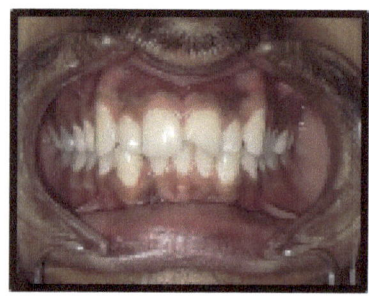

PRE OPERATIVE

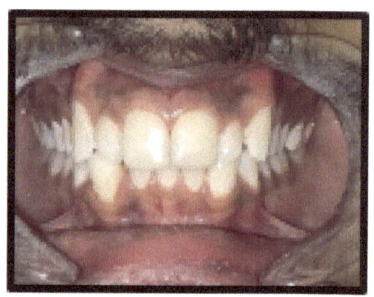

POST OPERATIVE

12

MANAGEMENT OF FRACTURED MAXILLARY RIGHT LATERAL INCISOR BY FIBER POST FOLLOWED BY CERCON (DENTSPLY SIRONA) CROWN

PATIENT NAME – Mayank

AGE/SEX – 22 Yrs/ Male

CHIEF COMPLAINT – Patient complains of broken tooth in upper front tooth region since 1 year.

HISTORY OF PRESENT ILLNESS – Patient gives a history of trauma 1 year ago.

INTRA-ORAL EXAMINATION – Ellis Class IV fracture irt 12

FINAL DIAGNOSIS – Ellis Class IV fracture irt 12

TREATMENT PLAN – Root canal therapy followed by fiber post irt 12

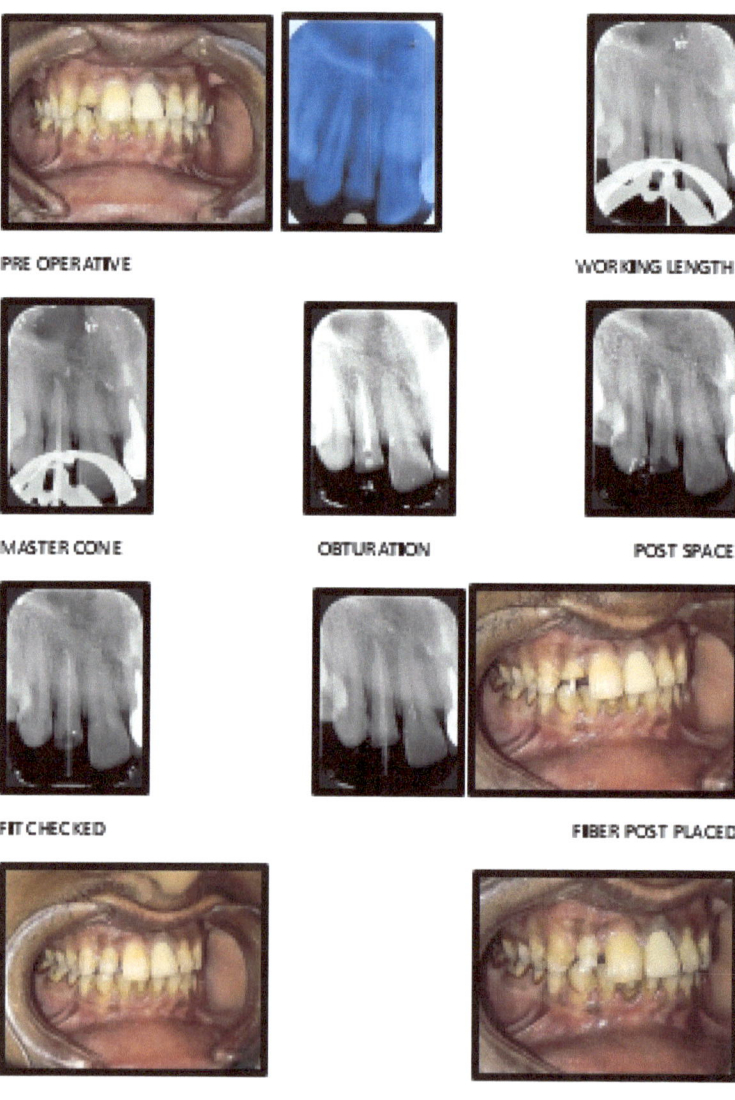

PRE OPERATIVE

WORKING LENGTH

MASTER CONE

OBTURATION

POST SPACE

FIT CHECKED

FIBER POST PLACED

CORE BUILDUP

CROWN PREPARATION

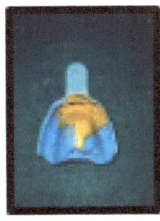

IMPRESSION

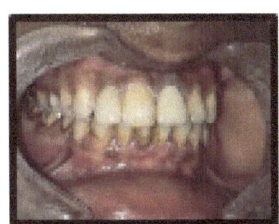

POST OPERATIVE

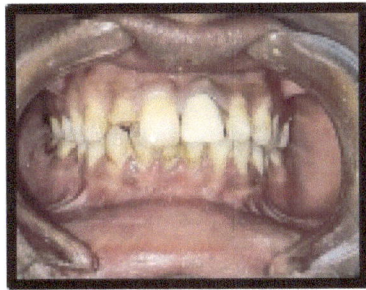

PRE OPERATIVE

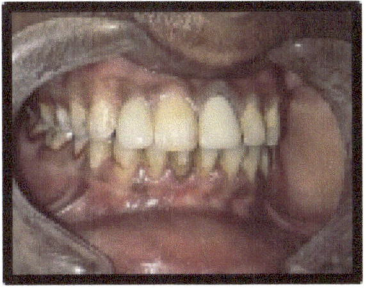

POST OPERATIVE

13

RETREATMENT OF LEFT MANDIBULAR FIRST MOLAR WITH FRACTURED INSTRUMENT BY BYPASSING IT

PATIENT NAME – Shayam

AGE/SEX – 17 Yrs/ Male

CHIEF COMPLAINT – Patient complains of pain in lower left back tooth region since 1month.

HISTORY OF PRESENT ILLNESS – Patient gives a history of RCT done in same tooth 2 months ago.

INTRA-ORAL EXAMINATION – Dislodged restoration, intra oral sinus opening irt 36

RADIOGRAPHIC EXAMINATION- Incomplete obturation, fractured instrument irt 36

TREATMENT PLAN – Re-RCT irt 36

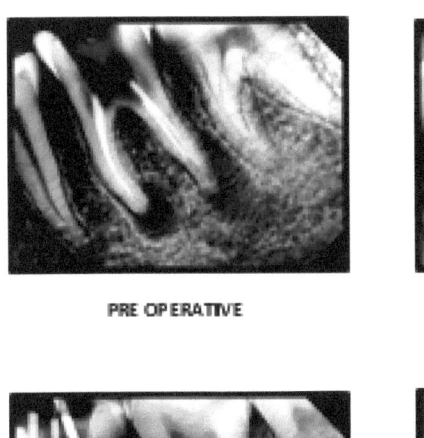

PRE OPERATIVE

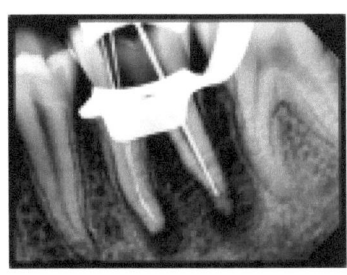

WORKING LENGTH

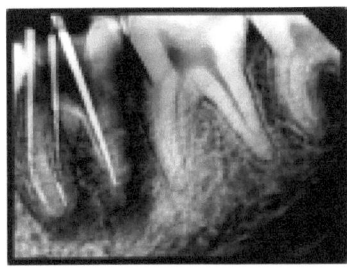

MASTER CONE

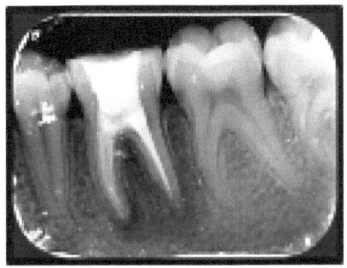

POST OPERATIVE

14

RETREATMENT AND FILE RETRIEVAL IN RIGHT MAXILLARY CENTRAL INCISOR FOLLOWED BY ZIRCONIA CROWN

PATIENT NAME – Anirudh

AGE/SEX – 21 Yrs/ Male

CHIEF COMPLAINT – Patient complains of pain in upper front tooth region since 1 month.

HISTORY OF PRESENT ILLNESS – Patient gives a history of RCT done in same tooth 5 months ago.

INTRA-ORAL EXAMINATION – Discoloured tooth irt 11, Ellis Class II fracture irt 21

RADIOGRAPHIC EXAMINATION- Incomplete obturation, seperated instrument irt 11

TREATMENT PLAN – Re-RCT irt 11

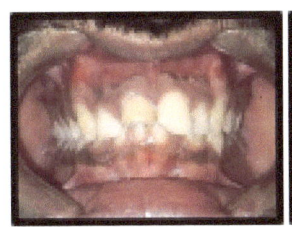 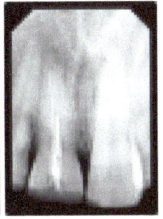 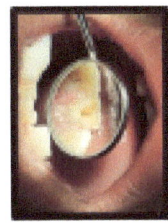

PRE OPERATIVE   SEPERATED INSTRUMENT

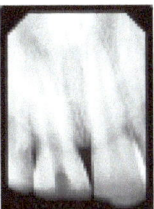 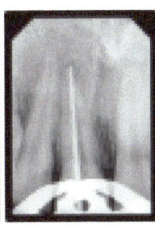 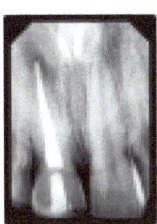

ROOT CANAL THERAPY

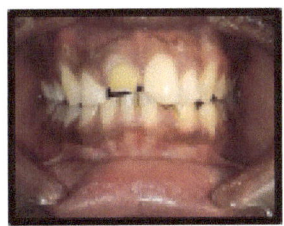 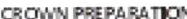 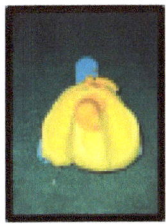

CROWN PREPARATION   IMPRESSION

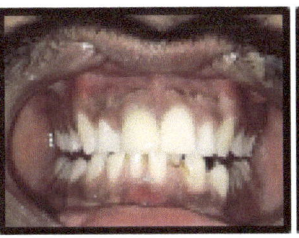 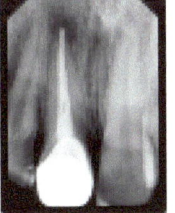

POST OPERATIVE

15

MANAGEMENT OF FRACTURED MAXILLARY RIGHT CENTRAL INCISOR BY CUSTOMISED FIBER POST AND CORE FOLLOWED BY PFM CROWN

PATIENT NAME – Shankar

AGE/SEX – 24 Yrs/ Male

CHIEF COMPLAINT – Patient complains of broken tooth in upper front tooth region since 5years.

HISTORY OF PRESENT ILLNESS – Patient gives a history of trauma in same tooth 5years ago.

INTRA-ORAL EXAMINATION – Discoloured tooth , Ellis Class IV fracture irt 11

TREATMENT PLAN – RCT followed by customized fiber post and core irt 11

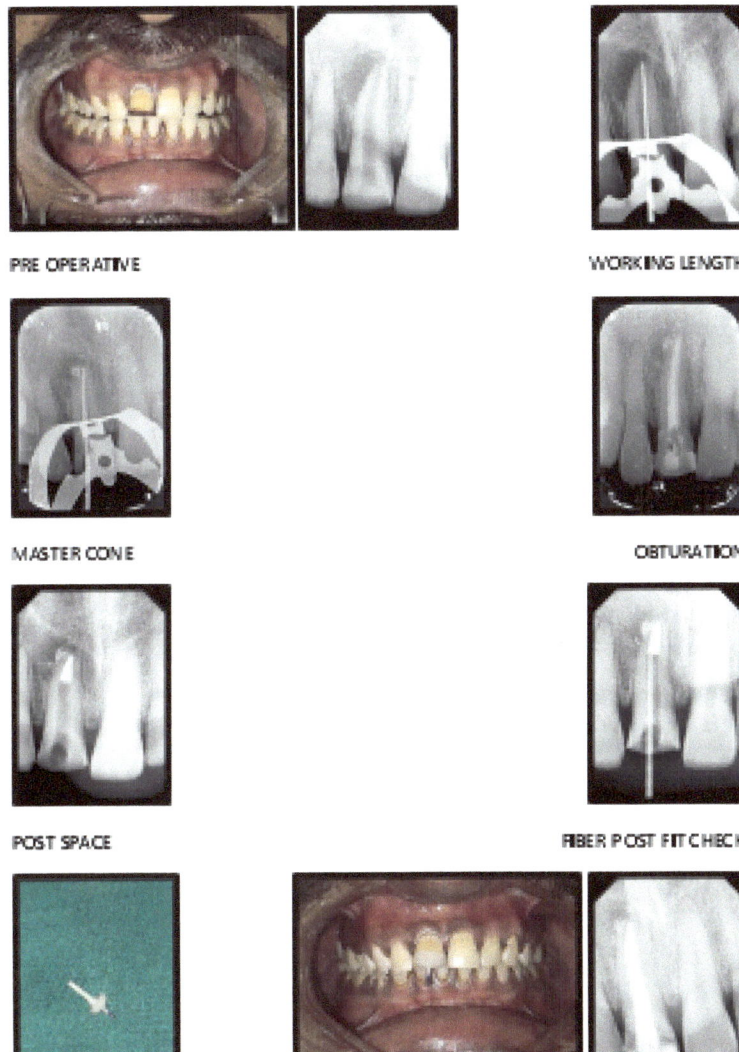

PRE OPERATIVE   WORKING LENGTH

MASTER CONE   OBTURATION

POST SPACE   FIBER POST FIT CHECK

CUSTOMISED FIBER POST AND CORE   CEMENTATION OF CUSTOMISED FIBER POST AND CORE

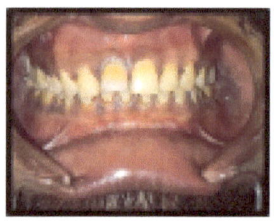
EXTRA FIBER POST REMOVED

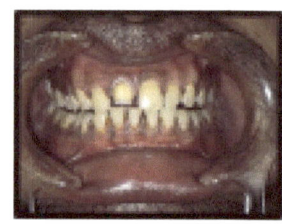
CROWN PREPARATION

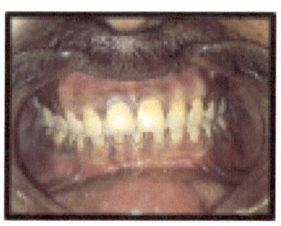
POST OPERATIVE

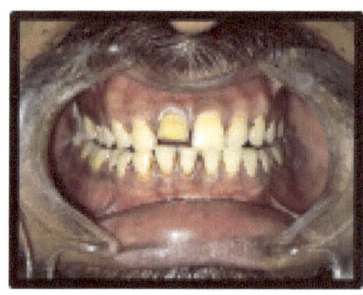
PRE OPERATIVE

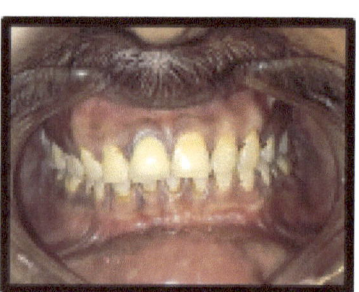
POST OPERATIVE

16

ESTHETIC MANAGEMENT OF ENDODONTICALLY TREATED RIGHT CENTRAL INCISOR WITH ELECTROCAUTRIZATION FOLLOWED BY ZIRCONIA CROWN

PATIENT NAME – Nitin Kumar

AGE/SEX – 34 Yrs/ Male

CHIEF COMPLAINT – Patient complains of broken and discoloured tooth in upper front teeth region since 8 years.

HISTORY OF PRESENT ILLNESS – Patient gives a history of trauma 8 years ago.

INTRA-ORAL EXAMINATION – Ellis Class IV fracture irt 11

FINAL DIAGNOSIS – Ellis Class IV fracture irt 11

TREATMENT PLAN – Root canal treatment followed by Electrocautrization and Zirconia crown irt 11

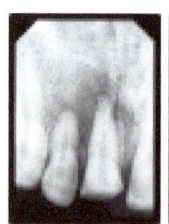
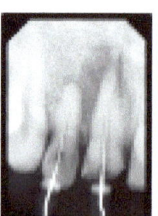
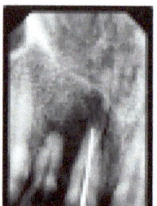
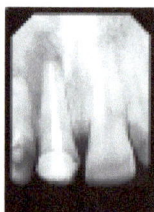

ROOT CANAL THERAPY

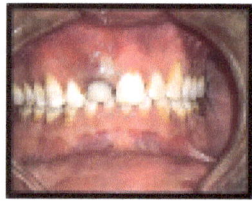
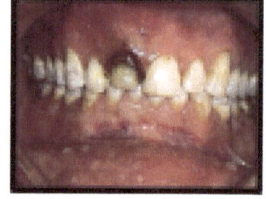

POST OBTURATION

ELECTROCAUTERIZATION

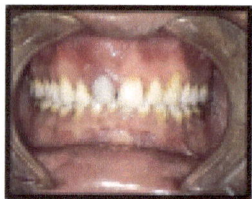
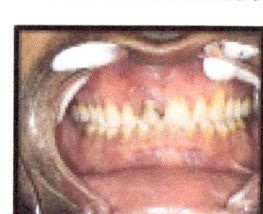

TISSUE HEALED

CROWN PREPARATION

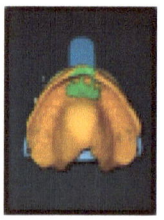
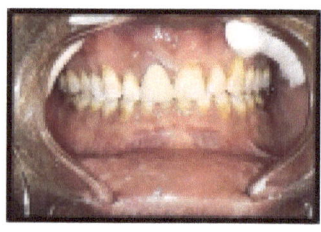

IMPRESSION

POST OPERATIVE

17

ESTHETIC MANAGEMENT OF ENDODONTICALLY TREATED MANDIBULAR LEFT FIRST MOLAR WITH CERAMIC OVERLAY USING CAD-CAM

PATIENT NAME – Ramesh Chand

AGE/SEX – 40 Yrs/ Male

CHIEF COMPLAINT – Patient complains of pain in lower left back tooth region since 1 week.

HISTORY OF PRESENT ILLNESS – Patient complains of pain in lower left back tooth region since 1 week.

INTRA-ORAL EXAMINATION – Dental caries irt 36, TOP +ve irt 36

RADIOGRAPHIC EXAMINATION- Radiolucency approaching pulp irt 36

FINAL DIAGNOSIS – Chronic irreversible pulpitis irt 36

TREATMENT PLAN – Root canal treatment followed by Ceramic overay using CAD-CAM irt 36

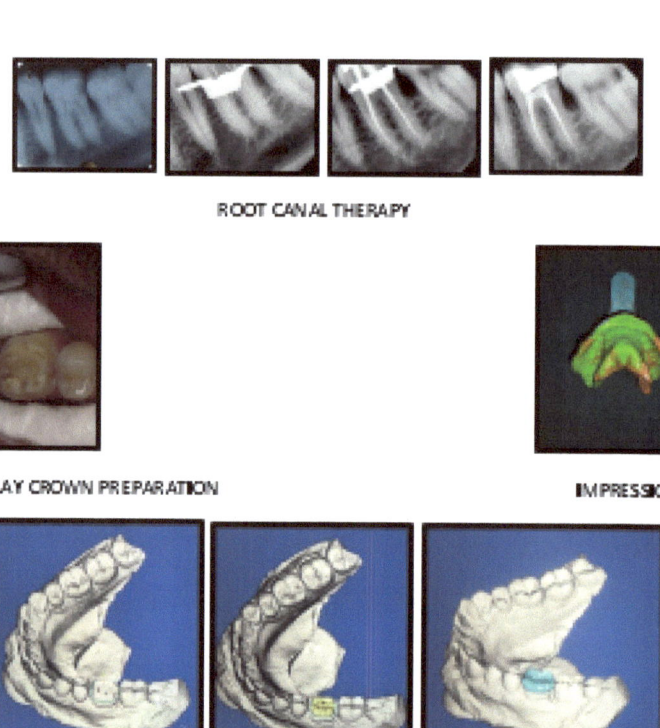

ROOT CANAL THERAPY

OVERLAY CROWN PREPARATION

IMPRESSION

CAD CAM

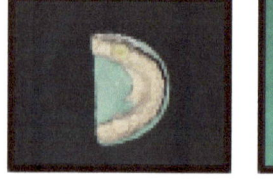

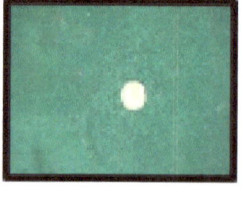

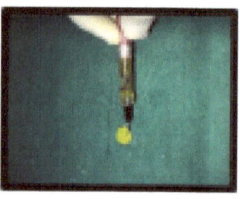

OVERLAY

INTAGLIO SURFACE OF OVERLAY

HF ETCHING

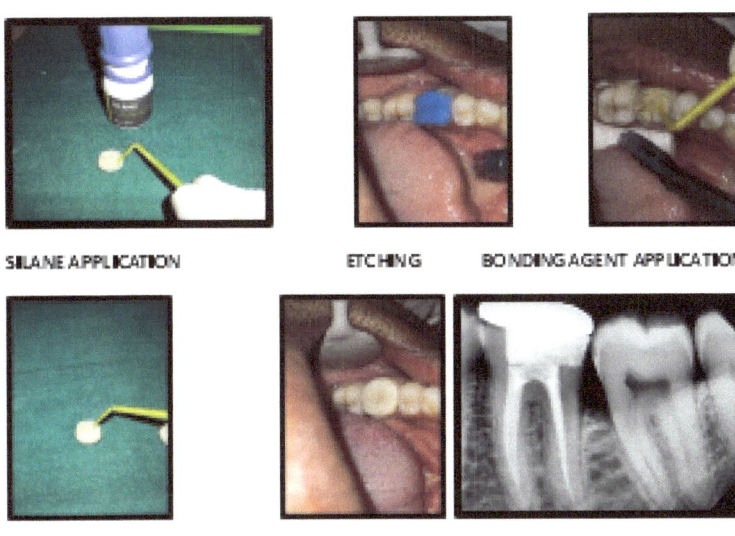

SILANE APPLICATION   ETCHING   BONDING AGENT APPLICATION

RESIN CEMENT   POST OPERATIVE

18

DIASTEMA CLOSURE IN MANDIBULAR ANTERIOR TEETH BY ENDODONTIC TREATMENT FOLLOWED BY EMAX CROWNS

PATIENT NAME – Yashoda

AGE/SEX – 20 Yrs/ Female

CHIEF COMPLAINT – Patient complains of gap in lower front teeth since 10 years.

HISTORY OF PRESENT ILLNESS – Patient complains of gap in lower front teeth since 10 years.

INTRA-ORAL EXAMINATION – Diastema irt 31,33,41,43; Missing irt 32,42

FINAL DIAGNOSIS – Diastema irt 31,33,41,43

TREATMENT PLAN – Root canal treatment followed by Emax crowns irt 31,32,41,42,43

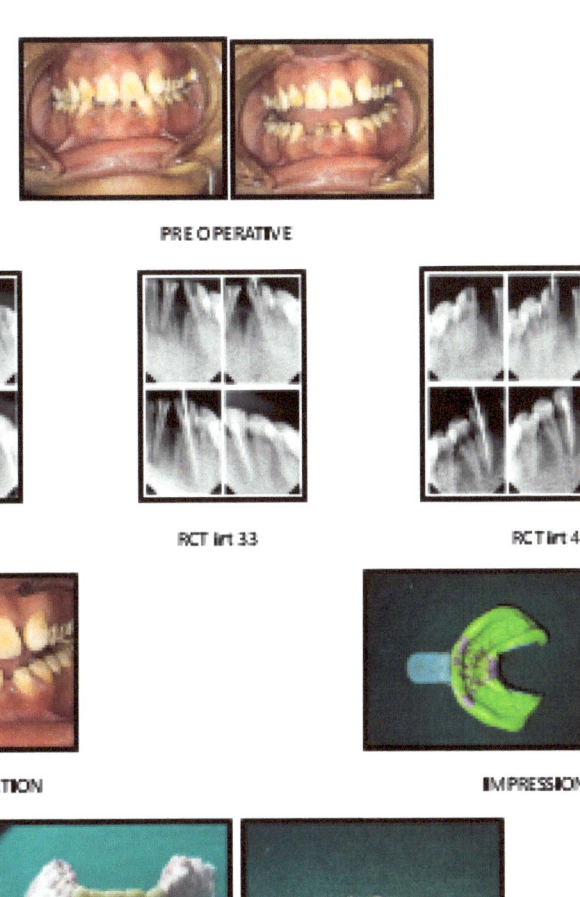

PRE OPERATIVE

RCT irt 31,41

RCT irt 33

RCT irt 43

CROWN PREPARATION

IMPRESSION

EMAX CROWNS

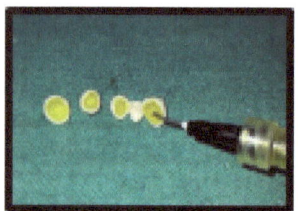

HF ETCHING

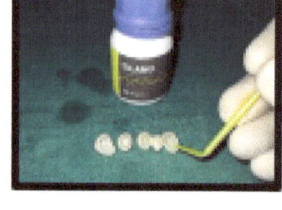

SILANE APPLICATION

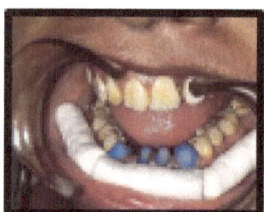

ETCHING

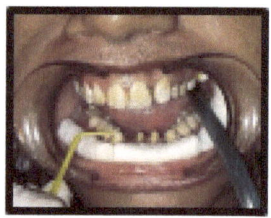

BONDING AGENT APPLICATION

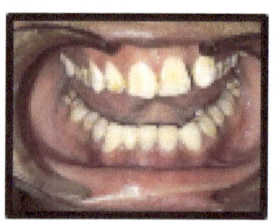

CROWN CEMENTATION

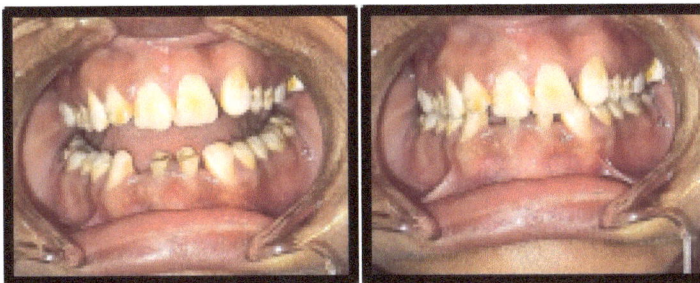

PRE OPERATIVE

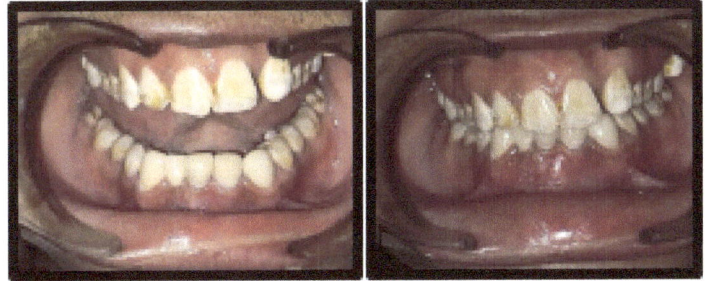

POST OPERATIVE

19

MANAGEMENT OF FRACTURED MAXILLARY LEFT CENTRAL INCISOR BY CAST POST FOLLOWED BY PFM CROWN

PATIENT NAME – Suresh

AGE/SEX – 20 Yrs/ Male

CHIEF COMPLAINT – Patient complains of broken tooth in upper front tooth region since 6years

HISTORY OF PRESENT ILLNESS – Patient gives history of trauma 6 years ago

INTRA-ORAL EXAMINATION – Ellis Class IV fracture irt 21

FINAL DIAGNOSIS – Ellis Class IV fracture irt 21

TREATMENT PLAN – Root canal treatment followed by cast post and PFM Crown irt 21

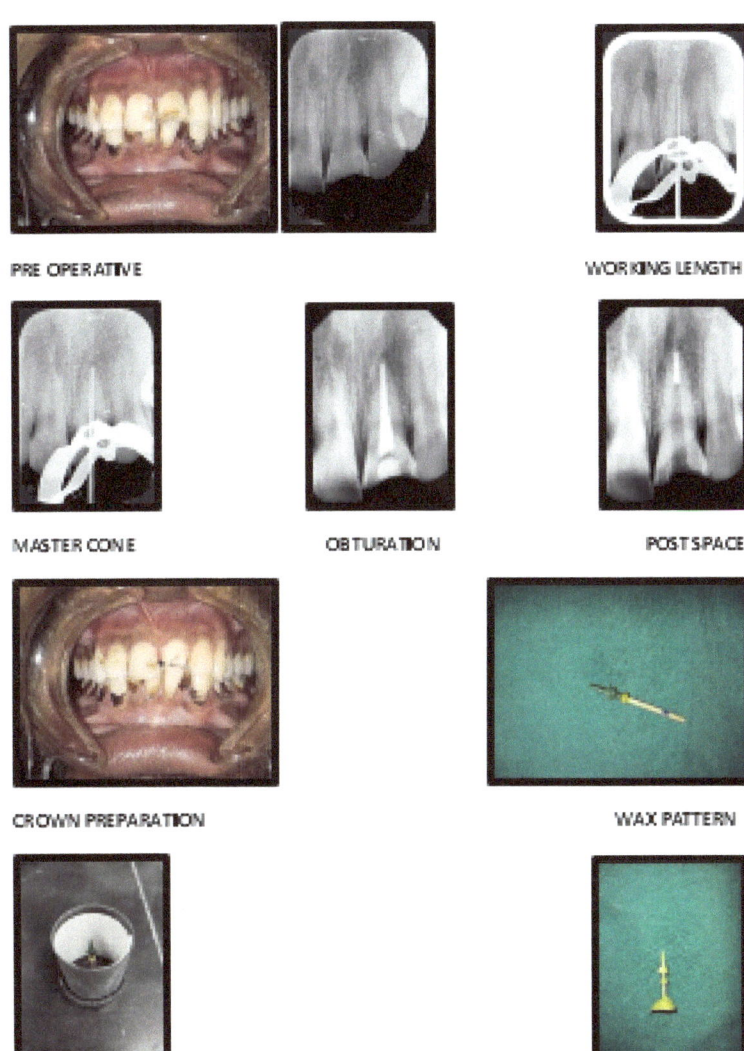

PRE OPERATIVE

WORKING LENGTH

MASTER CONE

OBTURATION

POST SPACE

CROWN PREPARATION

WAX PATTERN

INVESTING

CAST POST

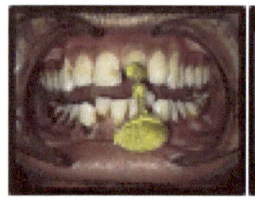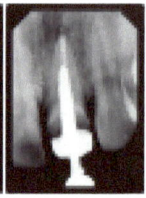

TRY IN OF CAST POST

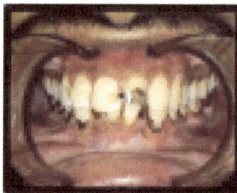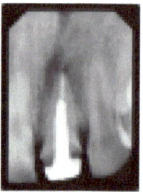

CAST POST CEMENTATION

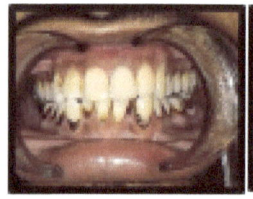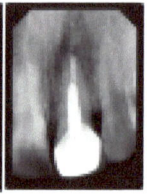

POST OPERATIVE

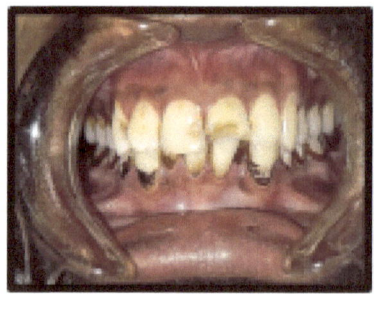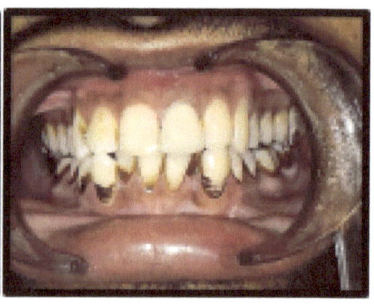

PRE OPERATIVE   POST OPERATIVE

20

ENDODONTIC MANAGEMENT OF RIGHT MANDIBULAR SECOND MOLAR FOLLOWED BY ENDOCROWN

PATIENT NAME – Mamta

AGE/SEX – 42 Yrs/ Female

CHIEF COMPLAINT – Patient complains of pain in lower right back tooth region since 10 days

HISTORY OF PRESENT ILLNESS – Patient gives history of filling in same tooth 10 days ago

INTRA-ORAL EXAMINATION – Fractured restoration irt 47

FINAL DIAGNOSIS – Faulty restoration irt 47

TREATMENT PLAN – Root canal treatment followed Endocrown irt 47

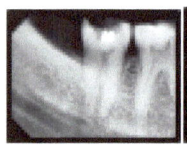 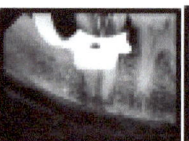 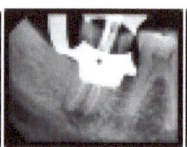 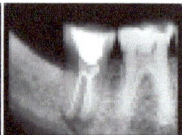

ROOT CANAL THERAPY irt 47

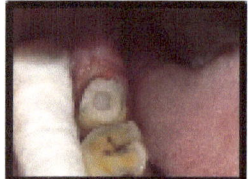

CROWN PREPARATION FOR ENDOCROWN

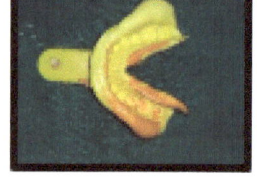

IMPRESSION

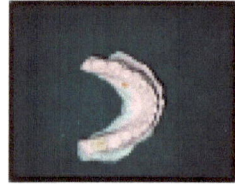 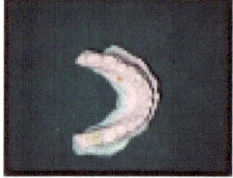

ENDOCROWN

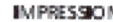

INTAGLIO SURFACE OF ENDOCROWN

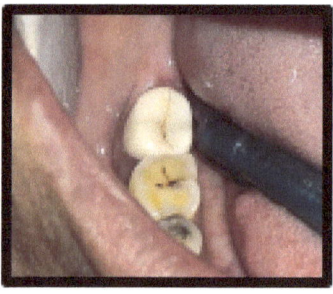 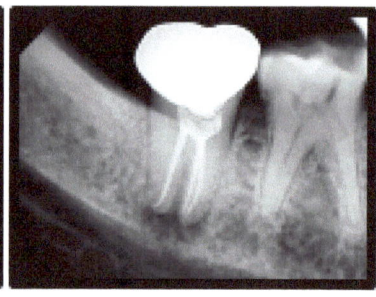

POST OPERATIVE